Fundoscopy for the MRCP

Fundoscopy for the MRCP

D. R. J. Jarrett MB BS MRCP

Senior Registrar in Geriatric Medicine, St Stephen's, St Mary Abbot's and Westminster Hospitals, London

M. L. Harris MB BS FRCSEd

Registrar in Ophthalmology, St Stephen's, Charing Cross and Westminster Hospitals, London

Churchill Livingstone 🏛

EDINBURGH LONDON MELBOURNE AND NEW YORK 1988

CHURCHILL LIVINGSTONE
Medical Division of Longman Group UK Limited

Distributed in the United States of America by Churchill
Livingstone Inc., 1560 Broadway, New York, N.Y. 10036,
and by associated companies, branches and
representatives throughout the world.

First published 1988

ISBN 0-443-03925-9

British Library Cataloguing in Publication Data
Jarrett, D. R. J.
    Fundoscopy for the MRCP.
    1. Man. Eyes. Fundus oculi. Diseases.
    I. Title.   II. Harris, M. L.
    617.7′4

Library of Congress Cataloging in Publication Data
Jarrett, D. R. J.
    Fundoscopy for the MRCP / D. R. J. Jarrett, M. L.
    Harris.
        p.   cm.
    ISBN 0-443-03925-9
    1. Fundus oculi — Diseases — Diagnosis —
Examinations, questions, etc.   2. Fundus oculi —
Examination — Examinations, questions, etc.
3. Ophthalmoscope and ophthalmoscopy —
Examinations, questions, etc.   I. Harris, M. L.
II. Title.
    [DNLM: 1. Fundus Oculi — examination questions.
    2. Ophthalmoscopy—examination questions.
WW   18   J37f]
RE545.J37   1988
617.7′3 — dc19
DNLM/DLC
for Library of Congress   87-36808

Produced by Longman Group (FE) Ltd
Printed in Hong Kong

Preface

Candidates in the clinical section of the MRCP examination
will have to examine the optic fundus — certainly in the long
case and possibly at least once in the short cases. Fundal
photographs also regularly appear in the slide section of the
examination. We have formed the impression, from our
teaching, that many candidates feel distinctly uneasy when
asked to comment on the appearance of the fundus. Most
medical textbooks give only a brief descriptive account of
fundal changes and usually fail to relate these to the
pathophysiology of the disease or the anatomy of the retina
and its adjacent structures. This information is contained in
the standard ophthalmological texts, but is often scattered in
such a way as to discourage all except the most diligent. We
have tried to cover — by the familiar format of questions,
answers and explanations, — most of the conditions likely to
be encountered in the examination and thus by practising
physicians. We hope this short picture book will also be of
benefit to undergraduates and any doctors who feel when
using the ophthalmoscope that they 'see as through a glass,
darkly'.

London   D. R. J. J.
1988   M. L. H.

Acknowledgments

Most of the slides used in this text were taken in the Ophthalmology Department of St Stephen's Hospital and we would like to thank Mr M. B. R. Mathalone and Mr R. P. Knowlden for their permission to use these.

We would also like to thank: the Medical Photography Department of Westminster Hospital for the illustrations to questions 26, 29, 30, 31, 32, 33, 34, 35, 37, 40, 45 & 46, Mr P. E. Kinnear for the illustrations to questions 39, 42 & 43 and also for his help in reviewing the text; Mr M. R. B. Mathalone for the illustrations to questions 27 & 28; Mr D. Taylor for the illustration to question 38; Mr J. J. Kanski for the illustration to question 47; Mr T. Rimmer for the illustration to question 15 and for his help in reading the text; Dr G. Fuller for his help in reviewing the text; the Medical Photography Department of St Stephen's Hospital for their help in preparing the photographs and illustrations.

Contents

Introduction   1

Questions and answers   11

Index   107

PART ONE

Introduction

Introduction

The direct ophthalmoscope was invented in the middle of the last century. In the last few decades, with the use of the electron microscope, the fundal changes in disease have been adequately related to anatomy and pathophysiology. A basic knowledge of the histology and function of the retina and its adjacent structures will clarify the understanding of most fundal abnormalities.

The eye develops from and around an outgrowth of neuroectoderm, the optic vesicle. This invaginates to form the double layered optic cup, the outer layer of which remains as the single cell layer — the retinal pigment epithelium (RPE). The inner layer develops into the multilayered structure known as the neurosensory retina. During development it is surrounded by blood vessels which later become the highly vascular choroid. The outer corneo-scleral layer develops from the surrounding mesoderm.

The adult retina is a transparent, inelastic, multilayered tissue. The outermost layer of the retina, the retinal pigment epithelium (RPE), is a layer of melanin containing cells with many functions, which include absorbing light and phagocytosing the photoreceptor discs as they are shed. They also provide essential nutrients to the photoreceptors (e.g. vitamin A) and form the outer blood retinal barrier. The finger-like processes of the RPE are in close apposition to the photoreceptor cells of the neurosensory retina. The potential space between these layers is where sub-retinal fluid gathers in retinal detachments. The outer segments of the photoreceptors contain membranous discs where the photoreactive pigments reside. Two types of photoreceptor cell are identified on morphological grounds: rods and cones. Rods are found throughout the retina and are responsible for scotopic vision (crude form vision at low levels of light). Cones are found in significant numbers only at the fovea and are responsible for photopic vision (precise daylight colour vision). Three types of cones are identifiable on the basis of their spectral sensitivity and they provide the sensory data for colour appreciation.

The remainder of the retina is composed of three nuclear layers and three fibre layers. The outer nuclear layer consists

4

Introduction

of the nuclei of the photoreceptor cells. The inner nuclear layer comprises the nuclei of the bipolar cells, the second neurones in the visual pathway, along with those of the retinal interneuronal cells (amacrine and horizontal) and glial cell nuclei. The innermost nuclear layer is the ganglion cell layer. The outer plexiform (fibre) layer contains the processes of the photoreceptor cells and the bipolar cells with which they connect. The inner plexiform layer contains the other processes of the bipolar cells and the dendrites of the ganglion cells. The innermost fibre layer is known as the nerve fibre layer and is composed of the non-myelinated axons of the ganglion cells. These run across the retina to exit at the optic disc where they are visible as the neuroretinal rim. As they pass through the sieve-like holes in the sclera (the lamina cribrosa) they become myelinated and constitute the optic nerve. These axons eventually synapse in the lateral geniculate bodies.

The retina has a dual blood supply. The inner retinal structures down to the inner nuclear layer are supplied by

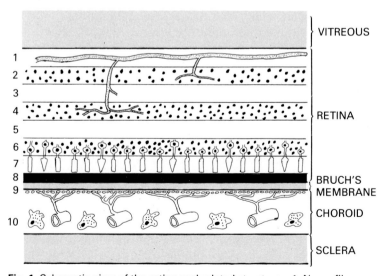

Fig. 1 Schematic view of the retina and related structures. 1. Nerve fibre layer with branches of central retinal artery (CRA). 2. Ganglion cell layer. 3. Inner plexiform layer. 4. Inner nuclear layer. 5. Outer plexiform layer. 6. Outer nuclear layer. 7. Rods and cones. 8. Retinal pigment epithelium (RPE). 9. Bruch's membrane. 10. Melanocytes and blood vessels.

Introduction

capillaries from branches of the central retinal artery. It is these arterioles which are seen with the ophthalmoscope as they run in the nerve fibre layer. The outer retina is supplied from the capillaries of the choroid (choriocapillaris) which form a vascular bed on which the RPE rests. As in the brain, the retina has barriers between the neural tissues and the blood. The inner blood retinal barrier is maintained by the tight junctions between the endothelial cells of the retinal capillaries. The outer blood retinal barrier is maintained by tight junctions between the RPE cells. Separating the RPE and the highly fenestrated choriocapillaris is Bruch's membrane. This is a thin (7 micron), laminated structure with a collagen/elastin/collagen sandwich between the basement membranes of the RPE and choriocapillaris. The choroid is supplied by the posterior ciliary arteries and drains to larger veins in its outer layers. The choroid also contains connective tissue and melanocytes. There is great individual and racial variation in the number of choroidal melanocytes which accounts for the varying background colour of the fundus. The choroid is the posterior portion of the uveal tract and is itself enclosed by the tough collagenous sclera. The retina, Bruch's membrane, choroid and sclera are schematically represented in Figure 1.

The optical system of the eye focuses the object of regard at the foveola. This is located two disc diameters temporal to and slightly below the centre of the optic disc. It is here that the retina is maximally thinned and consists of only tightly

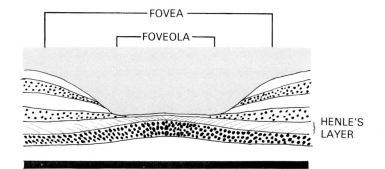

Fig. 2 Schematic section of the central retina.

Introduction

packed photoreceptors. It is only 350 microns in diameter and its blood supply is derived solely from the choriocapillaris, the inner retinal layers — normally supplied by the retinal vessels — being absent. This flattened area is surrounded by an area of retina with a sloping profile, the fovea centralis. The fovea is about 1.5 mm in diameter. This arrangement makes possible the high degree of visual acuity attained by the central retina. The fibres of the outer plexiform layer fan out radially from the foveola (Henle's layer), as shown in Figure 2. Surrounding the fovea the ganglion cell layer is several cells thick. The number of cells in the ganglion cell layer decreases with distance from the centre. Histologically the macula area is defined as the region where the ganglion cells are two or more cells thick, and is about 5.5 mm in diameter (Fig. 3). The macula region contains the yellow pigment, xanthophyl, from which its original name macula lutea was derived.

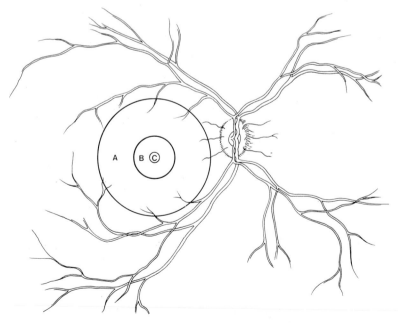

Fig. 3 A. Macula. B. Fovea. C. Foveola.

Introduction

The optic disc is the visible end of the optic nerve. It is oval in shape, with the long axis vertical and about 1.5 mm in diameter. It has a central depression known as the cup. The diameter of the cup is usually between 0.3 and 0.4 of the total disc diameter and should not vary greatly between the two eyes. Surrounding the cup is the pink neuroretinal rim of ganglion cell axons. The edges of the disc are usually easily identified, the nasal side being slightly less distinct than the temporal. The appearance of the disc varies with the refractive error of the eye. Hypermetropic eyes tend to have small optic nerve heads with consequent crowding of the neuroretinal tissue and loss of the central cup. Conversely myopic eyes have larger nerve heads and central cups. In addition the myopic disc frequently has a crescentic pale area with a pigmented edge on its temporal side, where the sclera is unmasked.

The retinal vessels emerge from the centre of the optic disc. The bifurcation of the central retinal artery is usually clearly visible unlike the veins which join deeper within the nerve head. The superior and inferior branches of the artery bifurcate again at or near the disc margin into nasal and temporal vessels. These four branches supply the four retinal quadrants, superior nasal, superior temporal, inferior nasal and inferior temporal. Venous drainage follows approximately the same pattern (Fig. 3). The arteries are narrower than the veins — the ratio of the diameters being about 2:3. The veins are darker than the arteries. Where the veins and arteries cross, the vessels share a common adventitial sheath.

The direct ophthalmoscope consists of a light, reflected into the patients eye by a mirror in the instrument's head. A small perforation in the mirror allows the examiner to observe the area illuminated by the light. Lenses interposed between the mirror and the examiner's eye are used to bring the view into focus. The power of these lenses can be changed by turning the knurled wheel at the edge of the instrument. In effect the dioptric power of the patient's eye magnifies the view of the fundus. The normal emmetropic eye has a power of 60 dioptres (D) and therefore gives an

Introduction

angular magnification of 15 × (Magnification = power/4).
The dioptric power of the myopic eye is greater than 60 D
and hence the view is magnified further, whilst in the
hypermetropic eye, with a lower dioptric power,
magnification is less.

It is best to take to the examination an ophthalmoscope
with which you are familiar. On all but the most basic
instruments there is a capacity for changing the size, colour
and other characteristics of the light beam. Narrow beams
are used for small pupils and larger beams for larger pupils.
Some beams have a grid pattern for measuring fundal
lesions, usually in comparison to the disc diameter. With the
red-free (green) source blood vessels appear black and small
vascular lesions are more easily seen. The slit-shaped beam
is used to show if a fundal lesion is flat, elevated or
depressed (Fig. 4).

When a good view of the fundus is required, the pupils
should be dilated, unless there is a history of acute
glaucoma, a shallow anterior chamber (where the iris seems
to be pressed up against the back of the cornea), or an acute
neurological condition where pupil size is of great clinical
importance. A short acting mydriatic agent such as

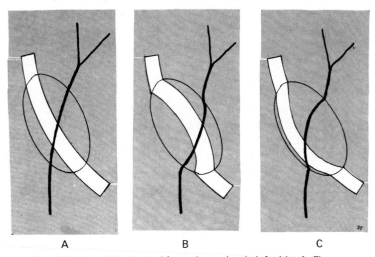

A	B	C

Fig. 4 Fundal lesions illuminated from the patient's left side. A. Flat.
B. Elevated. C. Depressed.

Introduction

tropicamide (0.5–1%) or cyclopentolate (0.5–1%) should be used. The fundus is best examined with the patient seated or semi-recumbent in a darkened room. From a distance of about 25 cm with a plus 5 lens a clear red reflex should be seen unless there is an opacity in the cornea, lens or vitreous. With total retinal detachment the red reflex is also lost. The patient's left eye should be examined with your left eye and his right eye with your right eye. Ask the patient to fix his gaze on a suitable point on the wall or ceiling. Rest your spare hand on the patient's forehead and if necessary the upper eyelid can be held open with the thumb. The ophthalmoscope should be held as close to one's own eye as possible to maximise the field of view. In practice it is easier to remove both your own and the patient's spectacles — the lenses in the instrument are used to correct your combined refractive errors. With a plus 5 or 6 D lens approach the patient's eye; having reached as close as you can to the eye, reduce the power of the lens in the ophthalmoscope head until the retina comes into sharp focus. By using this method you have brought the focus of the instrument through the optically clear media of the eye; cornea, aqueous, lens, vitreous and any opacities encountered should be noted. It is important to focus using the ophthalmoscope lenses rather than exerting your own accommodation. This may be made easier by pretending that you are peeping through the patient's pupil at an enormous distant fundus. Find a blood vessel and follow it back to the optic disc. Inspect the disc and then follow each of the vascular arcades out as far as you can. This is helped by asking the patient to look in the appropriate directions. Note the condition of the vessels and arterio-venous crossings as well as any lesions of the surrounding retina. Finally, inspect the fovea; this appears as a small bright round light reflex (as a general rule a bright light reflex is reflected from points of increased convexity or concavity, as at the fovea, from blood vessels or raised/depressed lesions). If you cannot find the fovea ask the patient to look directly into the light. In the clinical examination, as in clinical practice, politeness always makes a good impression, so thank the patient.

PART TWO

Questions and answers

Question 1

1. Name four abnormalities.
2. What is the likely diagnosis?

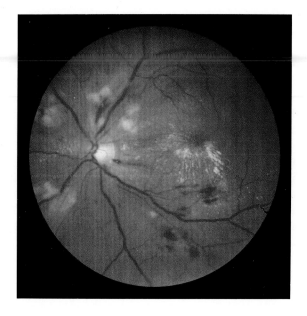

Answer to question 1

1. Arteriolar straightening, venous congestion, flame haemorrhages, cotton wool spots, and a macular star.
2. Accelerated hypertension.

The fundal changes in hypertension depend on its duration and its severity as well as the previous condition of the retinal vasculature. The initial response of the arterioles to hypertension is spasm, leading to thinning and straightening. The peculiar cytoarchitecture of the macula region, with the fibres of the outer plexiform layer (Henle's layer) running radially almost horizontally, makes it prone to accumulate oedema fluid. As the retinal pigment epithelium starts to pump clear the oedema, a protein residuum is left, seen as hard exudates between the fibres of Henle's layer giving the characteristic star appearance. With a severe rise in blood pressure the arteriolar constriction leads to retinal ischaemia characterised by cotton wool spots (previously misnamed as soft exudates) and flame haemorrhages. If unchecked, venous congestion and hyperaemia of the disc develop which may progress to severe disc swelling. Even with this degree of retinopathy visual symptoms may be absent. With effective treatment of the hypertension the disc swelling, haemorrhages and exudates resolve over a period of 6–8 weeks. Arteriosclerotic changes in the vessels remain.

Question 2

1. What does this show?
2. How would this patient present?

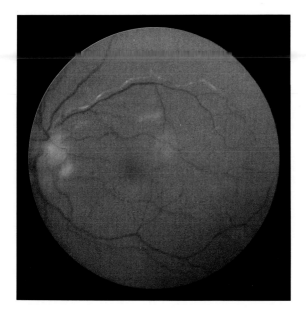

Answer to question 2

1. Multiple fibrinoplatelet emboli in the superior and inferior temporal arterioles (most marked in the upper) with cotton wool spots around the disc.
2. Painless loss of vision in the affected eye.

The macula area is supplied by branches of the superior and inferior temporal arteries and obstruction of one of these causes a sudden loss of vision often described as a 'curtain coming down'. This visual loss may be temporary (amaurosis fugax). In a small proportion of people the macular is supplied by the cilioretinal artery, a branch of the posterior ciliary arteries, and central vision may be spared. The ophthalmic artery is the first branch of the internal carotid artery and its branches may be occluded by emboli. Emboli may arise from:

Heart

Valves
— Vegetations (infective endocarditis)
— Calcific emboli (calcific aortic valve disease)

Chambers
— Mural thrombi

Major arteries

Cholesterol emboli
— These are yellow and glistening and often lodge at the bifurcation of arterioles

Fibrinoplatelet
— The usual cause of amaurosis fugax

Calcific
— Arising from the ascending aorta. They are usually large, single, white, irregular and located near the disc. They often cause permanent visual loss

Question 3

1. What is this condition?
2. Name four conditions with which it may be associated.

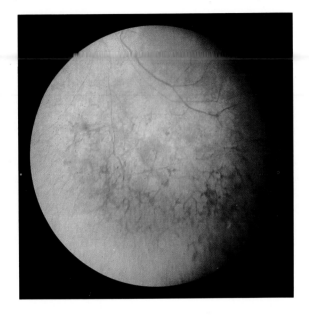

Answers to question 3

1. Retinitis pigmentosa (RP).
2. Refsum's syndrome, Friedreich's ataxia, abetalipoproteinaemia, Cockayne syndrome, Usher's syndrome, Laurence-Biedl-Moon syndrome, Kearns-Sayre's syndrome.

Retinitis pigmentosa is best regarded as a generic term for a group of disorders which result in dystrophic changes in the retinal receptors, predominantly the rods. The exact defect responsible in each type remains obscure. It may occur as an ocular disorder in isolation or as a manifestation of multisystem disease.

The ocular disorder may be inherited in an autosomal dominant, autosomal recessive or X-linked fashion. In general X-linked and recessive cases are more severe than dominants. Patients present with night-blindness and loss of visual field. The disease initially affects the mid-peripheral retina leading to the classical ring scotoma. Visible retinal changes are pigmentation in a bone spicule pattern, attentuation of the retinal arterioles, and waxy pallor of the optic disc. As the disease progresses the field loss becomes more severe and the underlying choroidal vasculature is revealed. Cataract is a common complication compounding further the visual difficulties. Genetic counselling is important. Unaffected carriers may be identified by abnormal electrical responses of the retina to light stimuli (electrophysiological studies).

Question 4

1. What is the abnormality?
2. How may it affect vision?

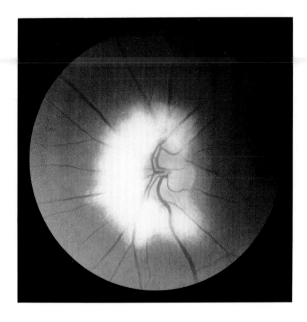

Answers to question 4

1. Myelinated nerve fibres.
2. Increase in size of the blind spot.

Myelination of the optic nerve fibres proceeds anteriorly
from the lateral geniculate body late in fetal development
and usually stops at the lamina cribrosa. In some people
myelination encroaches onto the fundus and appears as a
characteristic irregular pale fan of fibres radiating out from
the disc. Very rarely they extend out to the periphery of the
retina. Retinal vessels which run in the nerve fibre layer may
be obscured. They are of no clinical significance although
enlargement of the blind spot may be detected.

Question 5

1. What are these lesions?
2. With what conditions are they associated?

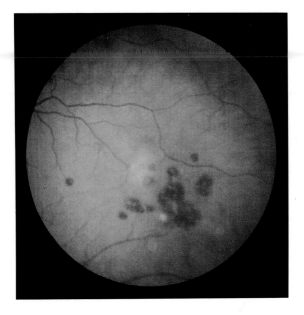

Answers to question 5

1. Roth spots (white centred haemorrhages).
2. Infective endocarditis, severe anaemia, leukaemia, anoxia.

Roth spots are small retinal haemorrhages with white centres. In infective endocarditis they are thought to represent an immune mediated vasculitis and occur in clusters; the number and position of the Roth spots varies during the course of the disease. In leukaemia the white centres are composed of leucocytes.

Question 6

1. What is the diagnosis?
2. What can predispose to this condition?

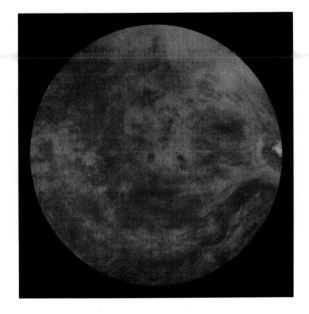

Answers to question 6

1. Haemorrhagic central retinal vein occlusion.
2. (a) Hypertension (70%).
   (b) Arteriosclerotic central retinal artery (compressing the central vein — they share the same adventitia).
   (c) Increased intra-ocular pressure (glaucoma).
   (d) Hyperviscosity syndromes — Waldenström's macroglobulinaemia, chronic leukaemia, polycythemia.
   (e) Periphlebitis — sarcoidosis, Behçet's disease.

In central retinal vein occlusion (CRVO) visual loss develops over a period of several hours. The retinal veins are dilated, there are haemorrhages all over the fundus, there may be cotton wool spots and the disc is swollen. Different types are identified by the number of haemorrhages and cotton wool spots. In venous stasis CRVO haemorrhages are less marked and there are few cotton wool spots. Prognosis for return of sight is better than in haemorrhagic CRVO which is more common in the elderly and in 20 per cent of cases leads to secondary neovascular glaucoma (in which the drainage angle between the iris and the cornea becomes blocked by neovascular tissue, resulting in a painful blind eye). This complication may be prevented by pan-retinal laser photocoagulation.

Question 7

A 35-year-old single man presents with vague constitutional upsets and a rapidly progressing visual deterioration in his right eye.

1. What is the diagnosis?
2. What one blood test would help confirm your diagnosis?

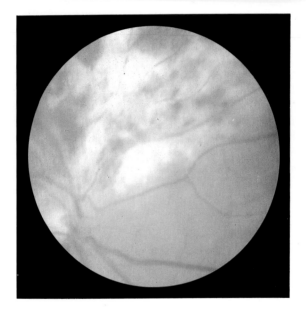

Answer to question 7

1. Cytomegalovirus (CMV) retinitis.
2. Human immunodeficiency virus (HIV) antibodies.

The appearance is that of CMV retinitis and the patient has acquired immunodeficiency syndrome (AIDS). The fundal appearance is said to resemble 'cottage cheese and ketchup'. The lesions may start peripherally or at the disc and rapidly spread along the vasculature. One or both eyes may be affected. The condition progresses rapidly over a matter of weeks resulting in blindness. There is no definitive treatment at present, but the acyclovir analogue gancyclovir has been shown to limit the progress of the disease. Other ocular features of AIDS include follicular conjunctivitis, dry eyes, Kaposi's sarcoma of the conjunctiva, herpes zoster ophthalmicus, anterior uveitis, multiple retinal cotton wool spots (50% of AIDS sufferers), toxoplasmosis, herpes simplex retinitis, candidal and cryptococcal retinochoroiditis.

Question 8

1. Name two abnormal features.
2. What can cause this appearance?

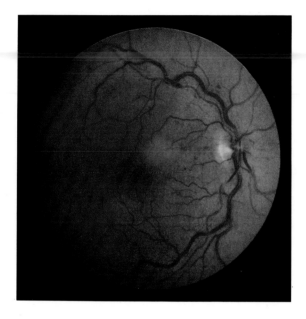

Answer to question 8

1. (a) Tortuous dilated veins.
   (b) Retinal haemorrhages — both superficial and deep intraretinal haemorrhages.
2. Hyperviscosity syndromes.

The retinal picture with hyperviscoscity of the blood includes dilated and tortuous veins, haemorrhages, cotton wool spots, microaneurysms and, if severe, congestion of the optic disc. Blood hyperviscosity may be caused by:

(a) Increased cellular components:
   Polycythaemia
   Leukaemia
(b) Increased plasma components:
   Waldenström's macroglobulinaemia
   Myeloma

A similar appearance of the retina may occur in carotid artery insufficiency (on the same side as the stenosis) and superior vena cava obstruction. Severe hyperviscosity may lead to central retinal vein occlusion.

Question 9

What does this show?

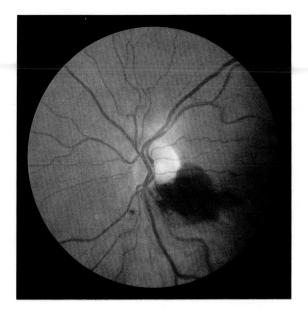

Answer to question 9

Retinal and pre-retinal haemorrhages.

The anatomical level of a haemorrhage can be gauged by, its size and its relation to the non-transparent retinal structures, namely vessels and the retinal pigment epithelium. If there is a relatively large potential space the haemorrhage will be large (preretinal, subretinal and choroidal). If there is little room for the blood the haemorrhages will be small as in deep intraretinal haemorrhages. In superficial retinal (nerve fibre layer) haemorrhages the blood follows the course of the nerve fibres giving them their flame shape.

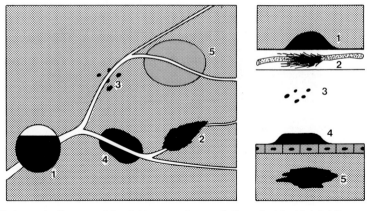

Schematic diagram of fundal haemorrhages. 1. Preretinal (subhyaloid) haemorrhages: large, often with a fluid level. 2. Nerve fibre layer haemorrhages: flame-shaped and obscure retinal vessels. 3. Deep intraretinal haemorrhages: small and deep to retinal vessels. 4. Subretinal haemorrhages: large and deep to retinal vessels. 5. Choroidal haemorrhages: large, deep to retinal vessels and grey (as deep to RPE).

Question 10

A young woman presented with an acute psychosis. She had a rash on her face and was anaemic. Her fundus is shown.

1. What is the predominant abnormality?
2. What is the most likely cause?

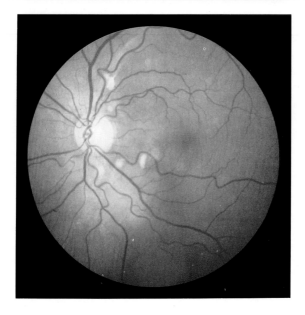

Answer to question 10

1. Multiple cotton wool spots.
2. Systemic lupus erythematosus (SLE).

Cotton wool spots represent areas of infarction in the nerve fibre layer. The axoplasmic flow along the axons is disrupted and the accumulation of cell organelles has led to the histological description of these lesions as cytoid bodies. They appear as white fluffy areas with an indistinct outline. Note that they obscure the retinal vessels and thus must be in the nerve fibre layer (see Question 9). They occur in hypertension, diabetes, retinal vascular occlusions, acute SLE, dermatomyositis, trauma, severe anaemia, Behçet's disease and AIDS — any process where there is retinal ischaemia. Cotton wool spots disappear if the underlying cause is treated.

Question 11

1. What is the diagnosis?
2. How is the patient's vision affected?

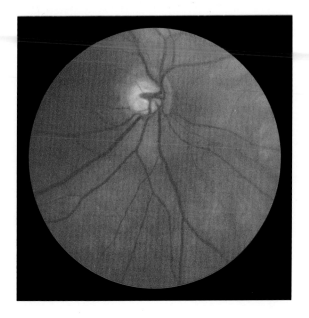

Answer to question 11

1. Chronic open angle glaucoma.
2. Visual acuity may be normal until a late stage, but the visual fields classically show an arcuate scotoma and constriction of the peripheral fields leading to tunnel vision.

Note that the optic cup is enlarged and extends to the edge of the disc which it never does in the normal disc. The blood vessels are displaced over to the nasal side of the disc and seem to emerge from its edge. Loss of nerve fibres leads to secondary optic atrophy (shown here). In early glaucoma vertical elongation of the optic cup is seen. Other signs are asymmetry in the appearance of the discs and small haemorrhages at the disc margin.

Question 12

A 21-year-old man presents with a 2 month history of
lethargy and joint pains. For 1 week he had noticed his gums
bleeding. His left fundus is shown.

1. Name two abnormalities.
2. What is the most likely cause of this appearance?

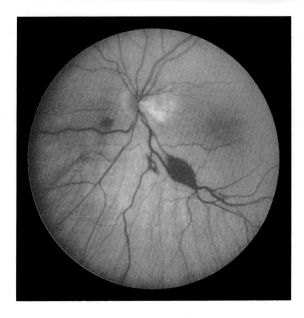

Answer to question 12

1. Roth spots and retinal haemorrhages.
2. Acute leukaemia.

About 50% of patients with leukaemia have some ocular involvement. The retinopathy is four times more common in acute leukaemias than chronic leukaemias. The characteristic picture is of intraretinal haemorrhages (although preretinal and choroidal haemorrhages also occur), Roth spots, hard exudates and cotton wool spots. Other features include tortuous veins (hyperviscosity) and perivascular sheathing with leukaemic cells. Micro-aneurysms and new vessels may develop in the peripheral retina. Leukaemic infiltration of the optic disc give rise to an appearance very similar to papilloedema. The different leukaemias are not associated with particular retinal lesions. During remission of the leukaemia the retinal changes resolve.

Question 13

A 30-year-old woman presents with a long history of intermittent headaches. She complained of no visual symptoms. It was noted that the retinal veins pulsated at the disc.

What is the cause of this disc appearance?

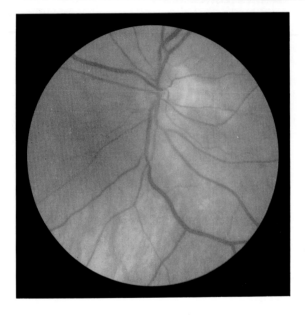

Answer to question 13

Pseudopapilloedema (hypermetropic disc).

Pulsation of retinal veins always excludes papilloedema. If this sign is not present gentle pressure on the globe will elicit it in the normal eye. A similar appearance may be seen in papillitis but in such cases there is a history of impairment of central vision. In hypermetropia the disc appears small due to:

(a) The whole eyeball including the disc being relatively reduced in size and
(b) The disc being less magnified when viewed through the less powerful optics of the hypermetropic eye.

The normal physiological cup is obliterated but the blood vessels are usually normal.

Question 14

1. Name two abnormalities.
2. What is the diagnosis?

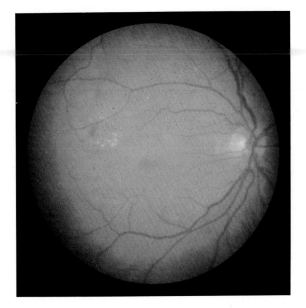

Answer to question 14

1. (a) Microaneurysms.

(b) Hard exudates — in circinate distribution.

2. Background diabetic retinopathy.

Venous dilation and microaneurysms are the earliest manifestation of diabetic retinopathy. Microaneurysms represent localised dilation of the venous side of the retinal capillaries. They are small, round with well circumscribed edges and are often located some distance from visible vessels.

Hard exudates are white and also have a distinct edge (cf. drusen) and are located in the outer plexiform layer of the retina. They consist of lipid laden macrophages — the result of leaking capillaries. They are often circinate (appear in a ring), forming at the edge of an area of leaking capillaries. In diabetic retinopathy they most commonly arise around the macula and are then termed focal exudative maculopathy. If hard exudates encroach on the fovea focal laser photocoagulation is required to close the leaking capillaries and reverse these changes.

Question 15

What is the diagnosis?

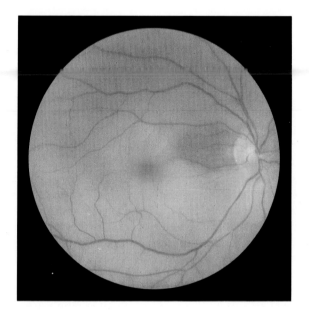

Answer to question 15

Central retinal artery occlusion (CRAO).

Central retinal artery occlusion presents as sudden painless loss of vision in one eye. An afferent pupillary defect (Marcus-Gunn pupil) will be present on the affected side.

The commonest cause of CRAO is thrombosis in an atheromatous artery. Large emboli, especially calcific emboli (see Question 2) can also cause this. Rarer causes include the arteritides such as giant cell arteritis (which more usually presents with ischaemic optic neuropathy), Takayasu's disease, the collagen-vascular diseases and Wegener's granulomatosis.

In the acute phase the retina is very pale (almost white) and oedematous. There is narrowing and irregularity of arterioles and venules and the blood columns may be segmented (trucking). Because the foveola is thinner than the surrounding retina the underlying choroidal vasculature becomes conspicuous — the 'cherry red spot'. In 5–10 per cent of cases the papillomacular bundle, or part of it, may be preserved — as is shown in this case — by the presence of a cilio-retinal artery. As the oedema resolves the normal colour returns to the retina but the vessels remain narrowed and secondary optic atrophy ensues.

CRAO is an ophthalmological emergency. Immediate treatment is aimed at re-establishing retinal circulation by:

(a) Intermittent massage of the globe; moderate pressure for 5 seconds being suddenly released for 5 seconds. This cycle is repeated for at least 15 minutes.
(b) Rebreathing of air, to increase arterial pCO_2 and cause vascular dilatation.
(c) Reduction of intraoccular pressure by intravenous acetazolamide and/or mannitol.
(d) In expert hands anterior paracentesis (release of aqueous under slit lamp control) can help.

The primary cause of the occlusion should be sought and treated if possible.

Question 16

This patient has had rheumatoid arthritis for many years. She was found to have bilateral central scotomas. Her fundus is shown.

What is the cause of her visual problem?

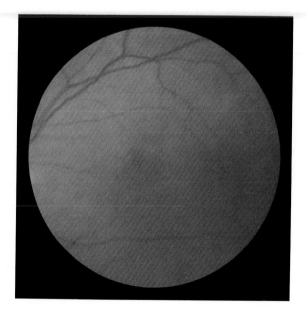

Answer to question 16

Chloroquine retinopathy.

Chloroquine, which is used in the treatment of rheumatoid arthritis and systemic lupus erythematosus, is strongly bound to melanin and reaches high concentrations in the melanin containing structures of the eye (the retinal pigment epithelium and the choroid). Retinopathy is rare in patients who have received less than 300 g total dose. Regular follow-up at 6 monthly intervals is required in patients on long term therapy to detect early signs of toxicity. The first visual abnormality is a central scotoma to a red target; the macula may appear entirely normal. Withdrawal of the drug at this stage usually prevents further deterioration.

In established maculopathy there is bilateral blurring of vision, loss of colour vision and central scotoma to red and white targets. There is loss of the foveal light reflex and fine pigment mottling of the macula. Bull's eye maculopathy (an early form is shown here) is rare and is characterised by perifoveal pigmentation surrounded by an area of depigmentation encircled by a rim of pigmentation. Established maculopathy is irreversible and can progress after the drug is stopped. In very advanced stages of retinopathy there is arteriolar constriction with loss of peripheral vision in addition to the central defect.

Question 17

This is the fundal appearance in a 75-year-old woman with normal visual acuity.

What abnormality is shown?

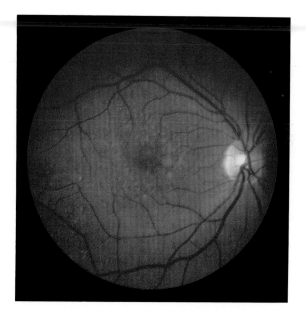

Answer to question 17

Macular drusen.

Drusen (colloid bodies) are small, yellow/white, discrete and slightly raised spots. They are common in the elderly and increase in size and number with advancing years. They are most numerous at the posterior pole (the macula) and are usually bilateral. They are the earliest sign of senile macular degeneration and visual acuity is frequently normal. Drusen are described as soft if the edge is indistinct and hard if the edge is sharp. Histologically they consist of collections of hyaline material lying between the retinal pigment epithelium (RPE) and Bruch's membrane, with atrophy and depigmentation of the overlying RPE cells and irregularities in the thickness of the underlying Bruch's membrane (see diagram). With time they may calcify and become 'hard' and shiny. There is evidence that soft drusen precede the development of senile disciform ('wet') mascular degeneration.

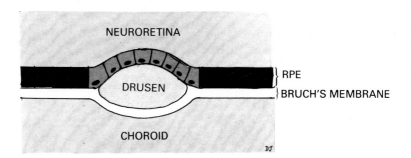

Question 18

This 45-year-old patient has been diabetic for many years.

1. What complication has arisen?
2. What further problem can result from this?

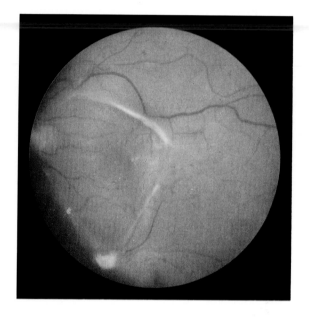

Answer to question 18

1. Preretinal fibrosis.
2. Tractional retinal detachment.

In proliferative diabetic retinopathy the neovascularisation is associated with fibrosis. The new vessels may regress with treatment but fibrosis may continue — the fibrous tissue becoming more dense and opaque with time. These fibrous bands radiate out from the disc to the vascular arcades. As the fibrous tissue shrinks, tractional retinal detachment may occur causing impairment of vision if the fovea is involved. Recently closed intraocular microsurgery with vitrectomy and division of fibrous bands has improved the chances of preserving vision.

Question 19

A 26-year old actress who has been diabetic since the age of 10 was noted to have this fundal appearance on routine fundoscopy.

1. What abnormality is shown?
2. What treatment is required?

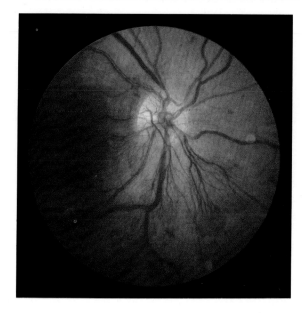

Answer to question 19

1. New vessels at the disc (NVD).
2. Panretinal photocoagulation.

Proliferative diabetic retinopathy is diagnosed when new vessels are detected on fundoscopy. These may be at the optic nerve head as here (NVD), or arising from other retinal vessels, most commonly the superior temporal vein (NVE — new vessels elsewhere). Proliferation is not limited to the retinal circulation, neovascularisation may be seen on the iris (rubeosis iridis). It is the most serious ocular complication of diabetes occuring in approximately 5% of all diabetics. Untreated it will cause blindness in about 70 per cent of cases within 5 years. New vessels at the disc have the worse prognosis. Initially the vision is normal hence the importance of screening for this disorder.

In proliferative diabetic retinopathy there is widespread retinal capillary closure and consequently ischaemia. Retinal hypoxia of any cause results in the release of an angiogenic factor leading to the formation of new vessels (neovascularisation). The neovascular tissue usually arises from the venous side of the circulation and appears as a network of delicate fronds. In contrast to normal retinal vessels the endothelial cells of new vessels lack tight junctions and are leaky. This can be shown by fluorescein angiography. New vessels initially lie flat against the inner surface of the retina. They are always associated with a fibrous tissue component although this is often not clinically evident in the early stages. The vitreous body contracts and pulls these fragile vessels forward, making them liable to rupture causing pre-retinal and vitreous haemorrhages.

When new vessels are seen urgent ophthalmological referral and treatment is required. Panretinal photocoagulation — treating the entire retina outside the temporal vascular arcades with argon laser or xenon arc light — reduces the production of angiogenic factor and the new vessels, but not the fibrous tissue, regress.

Question 20

This 74-year-old man presented with a history of recent difficulty with reading. The left eye had been lost in a previous industrial accident, the right fundus is shown.

1. What is the diagnosis?
2. What special investigation needs to be done urgently?

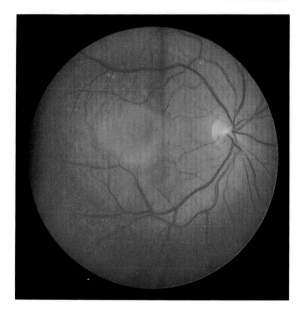

Answer to question 20

1. Serous macular detachment (exudative, 'wet', age-related macular degeneration (AMD).
2. Fluorescein angiography.

Rapid changes in vision are always significant at any age. In exudative macular degeneration, serous fluid in between the retinal receptors leads to symptoms of metamorphopsia (objects appear distorted) and micropsia\macropsia (objects appear smaller or larger than usual). The serous fluid is produced by exudation from subretinal new vessels which develop beneath the pigment epithelium, having grown through the Bruch's membrane often related to drusen. This leads to the typical dome shaped elevation of the macula seen here (note the distortion of the vessels as they cross the edge of the lesion). The area of the detachment is usually greater than that of the neovascular complex. Fluorescein angiography allows recognition of the subretinal new vessels and provided they do not encroach within 200 microns of the foveal avascular zone, laser photocoagulation can arrest the progress of the disease. Without laser treatment the eventual outcome is a fibrous disciform scar with destruction of the central retina.

Question 21

A 53-year-old woman with maturity onset diabetes melitus
was noted to have the lesion illustrated upon routine
fundoscopy. Her visual acuity was normal 6/6 Snellen.

What is the lesion demonstrated?

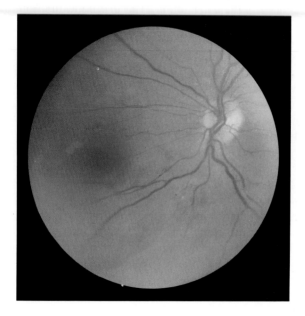

Answer to question 21

Benign choroidal naevus.

Choroidal naevi are common, occurring in 20% of the white population. They may be single or multiple and appear as round or oval, slate grey to blue lesions usually less than 3 disc diameters in size. They are flat or minimally raised with a hazy edge. They are present at birth and enlarge around puberty remaining constant in size thereafter. The lesions do not involve the choriocapillaris and the overlying retina is rarely damaged, although with the passage of time drusen may form. Macula lesions occasionally cause a serous retinal detatchment (accumulation of subretinal fluid without a tear in the overlying retina).

The lesion must be differentiated from malignant melanoma which appears raised and almost invariably leads to a serous retinal detachment with consequent visual loss. Malignant melanomas are often covered by small spots of orange lipofuscin pigment. Any enlargement in the size of a 'benign' naevus should raise the possibility of malignant change, although this is rare. In doubtful cases the size of the lesions can be followed by serial retinal photography. Fluorescein angiography and ultrasound scanning of the eye will also help to establish the diagnosis.

Question 22

A 62-year-old man presented with a 3 week history of blurred vision in the left eye. Further questioning revealed that it had come on over a period of 2–3 hours.

1. What abnormalities are evident?
2. What is the diagnosis?

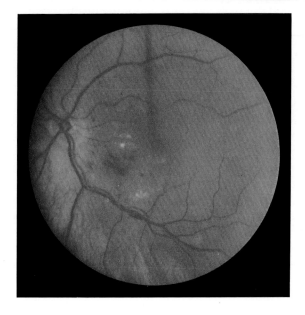

Answer to question 22

1. Flame haemorrhages, hard exudates.
2. Branch retinal vein occlusion.

Acute occlusion of a branch retinal vein will cause flame
haemorrhages, venous engorgement, cotton wool spots and
oedema in the area of retina drained by the occluded vessel.
As the oedema resolves hard exudates form.

The degree of visual impairment depends upon the vein
occluded. Vessels draining the fovea always cause marked
visual loss, whereas nasal or peripheral occlusions may pass
unnoticed. Visual symptoms develop over a matter of hours
rather than seconds, as is the case with arteriole occlusion.
Occlusion of one of the two main branches supplying the
central retinal vein leads to the superior or inferior half of
the retina being involved (hemivein occlusion). The cause is
compression of the vein at the disc margin, frequently seen
in chronic open angle glaucoma. Occlusions at arterio-
venous crossings are commonly due to hypertension and
arteriosclerosis. Peripheral occlusions may result from
retinal periphlebitis, inflammation of the veins, as seen in
Behçet's disease, sarcoidosis, and Eale's disease (retinal
periphlebitis of unknown aetiology typically occuring in
males of 30–50 years). Nasal vein occlusions have been
associated with diabetes mellitus.

Management involves treating any underlying cause. In a
proportion of cases capillary damage leads to large areas of
ischaemic retina and consequent neovascularisation. These
eyes may be identified by fluorescein angiography and laser
photocoagulation to the ischaemic area will prevent new
vessel formation and avoid the attendant risk of vitreous
haemorrhage.

Question 23

A 35-year-old Ghanaian woman was referred to the ophthalmology clinic when these lesions were noted by her optician.

What are these lesions?

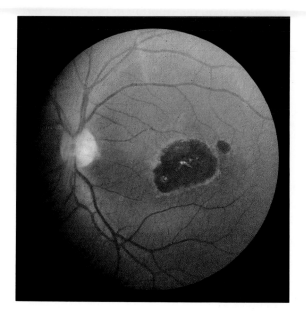

Answer to question 23

Inactive chorioretinitis most probably due to toxoplasmosis.

Toxoplasmosis is the most common cause of posterior uveitis in the Western World being responsible for up to 75% of cases. Toxoplasma gondii is an intracellular, protozoan parasite of widespread distribution in mammals, birds and reptiles. It seems likely that the majority of ocular infections are acquired in the first seven months of foetal life. The existence of adult acquired ocular infection is a matter of debate. Congenital infection can cause a range of abnormalities; most cases are sub-clinical but stillbirth, cerebral calcification, severe retinochoroiditis and microphthalmia may result. Ocular disease occurs in early adult life when dormant encysted forms of the organism reactivate causing seeding of the adjacent retina: 'satellite' lesions. The healed lesions have a pale central area of choroidal atrophy surrounded by a dark rim of hyperplastic retinal pigment epithelium (very marked in this case).
Other causes of posterior uveitis (choroiditis) include:

(a) Tuberculosis
(b) Syphilis
(c) Toxocariasis
(d) Sarcoidosis
(e) Behçet's disease

Question 24

A 70-year-old woman complains of gradual deterioration in vision.

1. What two abnormalities are shown?
2. What is the visual outcome?

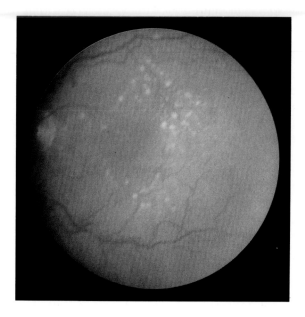

Answer to question 24

1. Drusen and atrophic macular degeneration.
2. Loss of central vision with retention of peripheral vision.

Drusen (Question 17) do not affect visual acuity per se. Senile macular degeneration — now more reasonably called age-related macular degeneration (AMD) — is the most common cause of blindness in the western world. Among over 65-year-olds it is the primary cause of visual loss in 40% of those registered blind. It is usually bilateral, and the incidence increases with age, 28% of 75–85-year-olds being affected.

Atrophic (dry) AMD is also known as areolar or geographical atrophy. The well circumscribed lesions represent areas of loss of RPE and overlying retina with variable loss of the choriocapillaris. Central and consequently colour vision are lost. Patients with advanced AMD retain peripheral, 'navigational', vision. There is no specific treatment for atrophic AMD, but patients may be helped by the provision of low visual aids (magnifyers and telescopic devices). Their home environment may be improved by high contrast labelling and point light sources rather than strip lighting.

In the United Kingdom a person is registered blind when they are 'so blind as to be unable to perform work for which eyesight is essential — in practice worse than 3/60 in each eye.

Question 25

A 16-year-old girl who has had type 1 diabetes mellitus for 10 years presents with blurring of vision in both eyes. The right fundus is shown. There is a similar appearance to the left fundus.

1. What is the diagnosis?
2. What is the treatment?

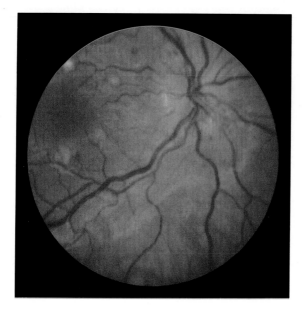

Answer to question 25

1. Diabetic papillopathy.
2. No specific treatment other than maintaining good diabetic control.

Diabetic papillopathy is a relatively rare complication of diabetes seen most commonly in young diabetics (teens and twenties). It is related to poor diabetic control and may be due to ischaemic damage to the posterior ciliary circulation supplying the optic nerve head. It is bilateral in 75% of cases. There is a variable degree of disc swelling which may be associated with capillary telangectasis, nerve fibre layer (flame) haemorrhages and macula oedema. Once good diabetic control has been re-established the condition resolves within a few months, although some studies report permanent visual loss.

Question 26

A 50-year-old man was admitted for inguinal hernia repair; he was otherwise healthy. The house surgeon was alarmed by the appearance of the optic discs, one of which is shown.

What is the diagnosis?

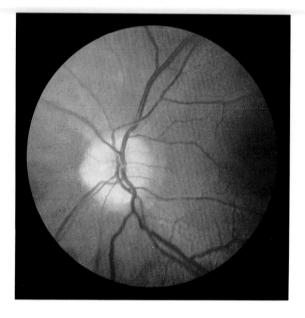

Answer to question 26

Optic disc drusen (hyaline bodies).

Optic disc drusen are often confused with papilloedema. They occur in 1% of the population, are a congenital abnormality and often familial (unlike macular drusen which are mostly degenerative). Initially they are buried in the nerve substance but become more prominent during adolescence. Optic nerve drusen are associated with visual field defects, arcuate scotomas and generalised constriction of the fields being commonest.

The following features are useful in distinguishing them from early papilloedema.
(a) Individual drusen give the disc margin an irregular notched appearance.
(b) Venous pulsation is present in 80%.
(c) The disc cup is filled in (crowding effect).
(d) The peripapillary nerve fibre layer remains distinguishable (seen here).

Disc drusen are associated with hypermetropia, retinitis pigmentosa and possibly with pseudoxanthoma elasticum.

Question 27

What is the diagnosis?

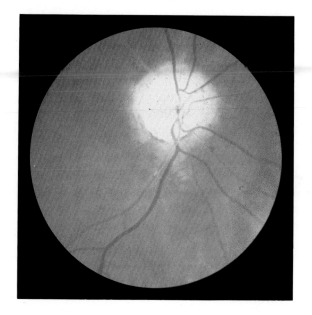

Answer to question 27

Optic atrophy.

Optic atrophy is caused by degeneration of the nerve fibre bundles of the optic nerve. The lesion may be anywhere along the course of the nerve fibres from the retinal ganglion cells to the lateral geniculate bodies. The nerve fibres lost are replaced by glial cell proliferation leading to the pale appearance. Loss of the retinal nerve fibre layer gives the disc a distinct outline. There is a variable degree of vascular attenuation.

Primary optic atrophy is a term applied when there has been no previous disc swelling. In secondary optic atrophy the disc has been swollen (papilloedema, papillitis, ischaemic optic neuropathy). The term consecutive atrophy is sometimes used for optic atrophy resulting from widespread retinal disease (retinitis pigmentosa, chorioretinitis).

Other causes of optic atrophy include:

Hereditary.

Leber's optic atrophy (an hereditary disorder affecting young adult males. It is bilateral although one eye is usually affected approximately 6 months before the other).
Dominant optic atrophy (an autosomal dominant condition, causing visual loss during the first decade of life). *Other disorders causing retinal degeneration* (e.g. retinitis pigmentosa, Tay-Sach's disease).

Acquired.

Trauma to the optic nerve (including birth hypoxia).
Infections (meningitis, encephalitis, neurosyphilis).
Demyelinating disorders. Pituitary tumours. Meningiomas (on the sphenoidal ridge). *Toxic* (methanol, quinine, tobacco amblyopia).

Question 28

This is the fundal appearance of a 22-year-old educationally subnormal epileptic.

1. What is the diagnosis?
2. What is the underlying condition?

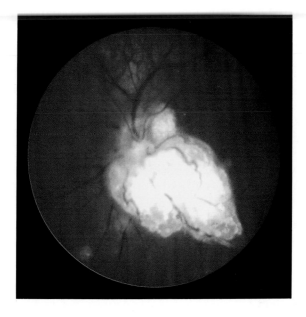

Answer to question 28

1. Retinal astrocytoma.
2. Tuberose sclerosis.

Tuberose sclerosis (epiloia, Bourneville's disease) is characterised by the triad of mental retardation, epilepsy and adenoma sebaceum. It is an irregular autosomal dominant condition; half of the cases occur sporadically. Hamartomas are found throughout the central nervous system. In 50% retinal astrocytomas are present. They occur most commonly at or around the optic disc and usually appear as well circumscribed nodular lesions. With time multiple areas of calcification develop giving rise to the 'mulberry' appearance as shown. They are usually asymptomatic and very slow growing.

Tuberose sclerosis is one of the phakomatoses; this is a group of hereditary conditions where neurological abnormalities are associated with skin, retinal and other changes. The four main groups are:

(a) Neurofibromatosis
— multiple neurofibromas, café au lait spots, bone abnormalities, etc.
(b) Sturge-Weber syndrome
— cutaneous angioma in the distribution of the trigeminal nerve, meningeal angiomas, choroidal angiomas causing secondary glaucoma
(c) Von Hippel-Lindau syndrome
— retinal angiomas, cysts and tumours of the cerebellum and abdominal organs
(d) Tuberose sclerosis

Question 29

A 28-year-old woman was admitted to hospital with haematemesis and melaena. Her fundus is shown.

1. What abnormality is present?
2. What is the underlying condition?

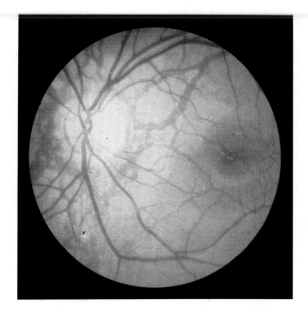

Answer to question 29

1. Angioid streaks.
2. Pseudoxanthoma elasticum.

Pseudoxanthoma elasticum is a hereditary disorder, usually autosomal recessive, although dominant transmission has been described. It affects the skin, eyes, and small arteries. The precise pathology is uncertain but there is a defect in elastin. The skin changes range from yellow papules, most commonly found in the neck, axilla and antecubital fossa, to larger plaques causing redundant skin folds. Involvement of the media of small arteries causes bleeding from the gut, uterus and other organs.

Angioid streaks occur in all but a few cases and are usually bilateral. They represent breaks in Bruch's membrane and appear as dark red or grey flat lines most marked around the disc. They run under the retinal vessels and can be further differentiated from veins by their irregular edge, bizarre pattern and greater size. Other causes of angioid streaks are:

(a) Idiopathic
(b) Paget's disease of bone
(c) Ehlers-Danlos syndrome
(d) Sickle cell disease

Question 30

A 50-year-old man was referred to the ophthalmology clinic because of this abnormal disc appearance.

1. What abnormality is shown?
2. What is the significance?

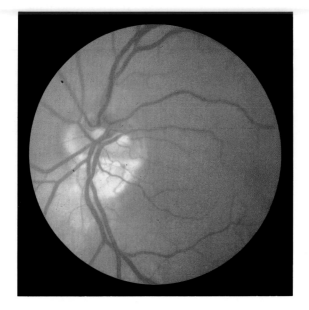

Answer to question 30

1. Tilted disc.
2. Possible cause of visual field defects.

The normal disc is oval in shape with the long axis vertical. In tilted discs the optic nerve enters the eye at an oblique angle. This condition is relatively common and usually bilateral. Corrected visual acuity is normal (myopia and astigmatism are common). It is not associated with any systemic disorders. Hypopigmentation of the inferior nasal retina often occurs and gives rise to an upper temporal field defect. The field changes are not strictly related to the vertical midline allowing differentiation from the bitemporal hemianopia of chiasmal compression.

Question 31

A young man presents with a history of headaches and vomiting. On further questioning he complains of episodic loss of vision lasting a few seconds at a time.

1. What fundal abnormality is shown?
2. What visual field defect is likely?

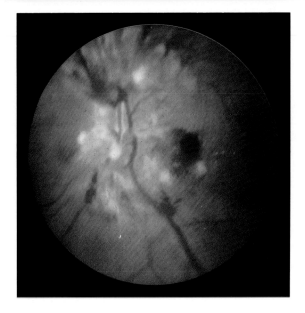

Answer to question 31

1. Established papilloedema.
2. Enlarged blind spot and concentric constriction of the visual fields.

There are many causes of a swollen optic nerve head; the term papilloedema is reserved for cases where the swelling is due to raised intracranial pressure.

In established papilloedema the disc margins are lost and the central cup obliterated. The veins are engorged; haemorrhages and cotton wool spots are present. The nerve head is elevated above the retina which may show concentric folds as here. Haemorrhages and cotton wool spots are more marked in papilloedema of rapid onset. Transient obscurations of vision are typical of severe papilloedema, possibly due to temporary impairment of retinal blood flow. They carry a poor visual prognosis signalling the onset of secondary optic atrophy. Enlargement of the blind spot is the commonest visual field defect in papilloedema, the extent is variable but when the raised intracranial pressure has been present for a period of months the enlargement may mimic bitemporal hemianopia. Generalised constriction of the field is also seen.

The causes of raised intracranial pressure include:

(a) Space occupying lesions — tumours, abcesses etc. (especially in the fourth ventricle, cerebellum and temporal lobes).
(b) Meningitis.
(c) Benign intracranial hypertension.

Question 32

A 25-year-old woman complains of recent onset of blurred vision in a 'lazy' eye.

What is the diagnosis?

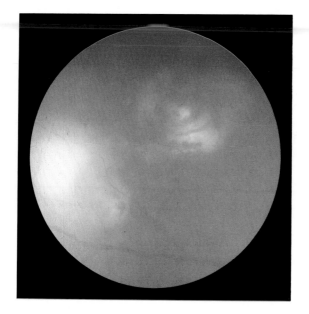

Answer to question 32

Active toxoplasma choroiditis.

The photograph shows a healed choroiditis lesion over the fovea, probably congenital and the cause of her amblyopic (lazy) eye. There is also an active satellite lesion causing the recent change in vision. The active disease is characterised by pale pink to white, slightly raised lesions with an indistinct edge, most commonly in the posterior pole. The disease is self limiting and treatment is only indicated if the fovea or optic nerve are threatened. Treatment is with sulphonamides ('Triple sulpha') and pyrimethamine or clindamycin. Oral steroids are often used in combination with either of these regimes. Encysted forms are not destroyed by treatment and further reactivation may ensue.

Question 33

How would you describe this fundal appearance?

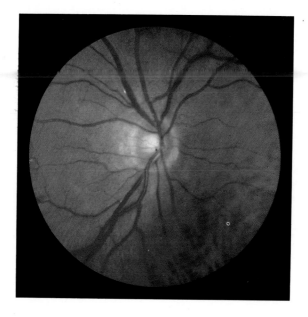

Answer to question 33

Tigroid fundus.

The background colour of the fundus depends on the amount and distribution of melanocytes in the choroid. Usually there is even distribution but in some dark skinned or dark haired people it is uneven. This gives rise to a tigroid appearance. It is of no pathological significance.

Question 34

A 70-year-old man complains of recent loss of vision in the right eye.

What is the diagnosis?

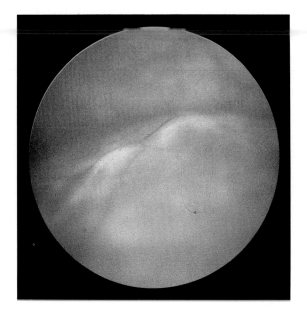

Answer to question 34

Malignant melanoma of the choroid.

Malignant melanoma of the choroid is the commonest primary intraocular tumour in the adult. They appear as raised oval masses with a varying degree of pigmentation, usually brown or dark grey. Amelanotic melanomas do occur and may be difficult to distinguish from choroidal secondaries. They are most common at the posterior pole but may involve any part of the uveal tract (iris, ciliary body and choroid). Presentation depends upon the site and size of the lesion. With posterior uveal lesions field loss occurs due to the overlying serous retinal detachment, when the foveal area becomes involved there is loss of visual acuity and metamorphopsia. Ocular transillumination, ultrasonography and fluorescein angiography help to confirm the diagnosis. The most common sites of metastases are the liver and lungs.

The treatment of choroidal malignant melanomas is a controversial subject. In the past enucleation was regarded as mandatory. The choice nowadays is between enucleation, local radioactive plaques, external beam radiotherapy, local excision, photocoagulation and regular observation; this depends upon the age of the patient, the tumour size, the visual acuity, the presence of pain and metastatic disease.

Question 35

What two abnormalities are shown?

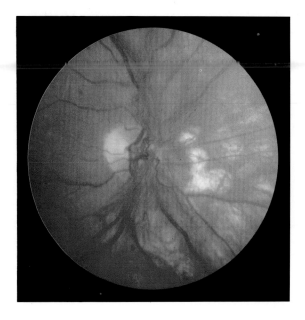

Answer to question 35

(a) New vessels at the disc (NVD).
(b) Photocoagulation scars.

Fresh photocoagulation scars appear white with an indistinct edge. As healing occurs they acquire a rim of pigment and the underlying choroidal vasculature may be revealed (cf. healed choroiditis). The energy of the laser light is absorbed by the pigments in the retina, especially the retinal pigment epithelium. A thermal burn results involving the outer retinal layers. In proliferative diabetic retinopathy multiple laser burns are applied to the entire retinal periphery (2000–3000 individual burns). This reduces the production of angiogenic factor and reverses the neovascular process. In the treatment of diabetic maculopathy the laser burns seal leaking vessels and stimulate the RPE cells to clear retinal oedema. In focal exudative maculopathy the laser is applied to the centre of the circinate lesions. In cystoid maculopathy, where there is diffuse macula oedema, treatment consists of applying a grid pattern of laser burns surrounding the fovea to clear the oedema, but the visual results are often disappointing.

Question 36

How would you describe the appearance of this disc?

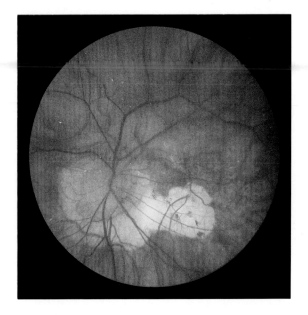

Answer to question 36

Myopic disc.

In myopia the axial length of the eye is increased. The retina is inelastic and with lengthening of the eyeball the sclera is exposed which appears as the white myopic crescent, often rimmed with pigment. This is usually on the temporal side of the disc but may be seen as an annular ring as in this case. On ophthalmoscopy the disc and retina appear larger than in the emmetropic patient (see introduction).

Simple myopia is very common and does not lead to complications. In higher degrees of myopia (>6 dioptres) chorioretinal degeneration can occur. This degenerative process is not restricted to the disc margin, but can spread across the posterior pole. Atrophy of the RPE and choriocapillaris leads to the white appearance of these lesions which display a variable degree of marginal pigmentation. Breaks in Bruch's membrane and haemorrhages may also occur. The exact pathology of these lesions is unclear. In addition high myopes have a greater incidence of peripheral retinal degenerations and as a consequence are prone to rhegmatogenous retinal detatchments (tears or holes in the retina allow fluid into the subretinal space).

Question 37

A 35-year-old man is found wandering in the street. He is unable to give a clear account of himself. The left plantar response is extensor. Both fundi have a similar appearance.

What does this fundus show?

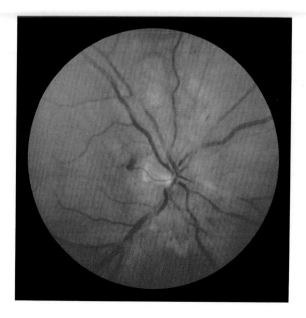

Answer to question 37

Papilloedema.

The optic nerve is surrounded by meninges and CSF for its entire length. With raised intracranial pressure of any cause the increased pressure is conducted to the optic nerve. This causes papilloedema by two possible mechanisms.
Vascular. The veins draining the optic nerve head pass through the subarachnoid space. In raised intracranial pressure venous return is impaired and disc oedema results.
Mechanical. Compression of the nerves impairs axoplasmic flow leading to leakage of fluid, protein and cytoplasmic constituents. This leads to osmotically induced swelling.
   In papilloedema visible changes in the vascular and nervous tissue of the disc are seen. Early vascular signs are hyperaemia, venous engorgement, increased tortuosity and loss of venous pulsation. If venous pulsation is seen papilloedema can be excluded, but its absence does not necessarily imply raised intracranial pressure. The earliest neural changes are blurring of the nasal, superior and inferior disc margins. The optic cup is preserved until late. As the papilloedema progresses the temporal margin is lost and the nerve head rises above the retinal surface causing concentric folds in the surrounding choroid and retina. The congested vessels seem to disappear as they enter the indistinct disc edge which is encircled by haemorrhages and exudates. The height of the disc elevation can be given a dioptric value by noting the power of lens required to focus on the nerve head and comparing this to that required to focus on the retinal surface. Readings are taken by counting the number of clicks between each focus then referring to the lens powers displayed on the ophthalmoscope head. Despite these changes visual acuity remains normal, unless secondary optic atrophy occurs pressaged by transient obscurations of vision.
   After relief of the raised intracranial pressure papilloedema takes 6–8 weeks to resolve.

Question 38

1. What abnormality is shown?
2. With what conditions is it associated?

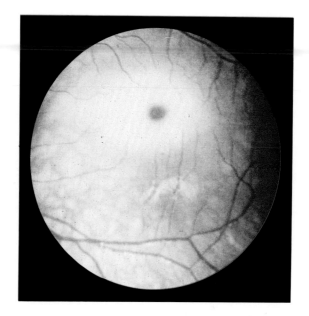

Answer to question 38

1. Cherry red spot.
2. Neuronal storage diseases:
  (a) Tay-Sachs disease
  (b) Niemann-Pick disease
  (c) Sandhoff's disease
  (d) Sialidosis
  (e) Infantile Gm1 gangliosidosis
  (f) Late onset Gm2 gangliosidosis

The neurolipidoses (neuronal storage diseases) comprise a number of rare, usually autosomal recessive, inborn errors of metabolism. They result in the intracellular deposition of phospholipids or glycolipids. When the retina is involved lipids are deposited in the ganglion cell layer and give it a pale appearance. As the foveola has no ganglion cell layer the underlying choroidal vasculature appears bright red in contrast to the rest of the macula with its thicker layer of ganglion cells. This gives rise to the 'cherry red spot' picture. Later in the course of the diseases the gangliion cells and subsequently the nerve fibre layer is destroyed and optic atrophy results.

Tay-Sachs (Gm2-gangliosidosis type 1) is the commonest of these conditions and results from the deficiency of the lysosomal enzyme hexosaminidase. The disease starts in the first year of life with visual loss, progressive neurological deterioration and spasticity. 90% of cases have a cherry red spot. Survival after the age of 4 years is rare.

In Niemann-Pick disease there is deficiency of sphyngomyelinase with accumulation of sphyngomyelin. Two types are recognised. In type A (85% of cases) the central nervous system is involved; the cherry red spot is found less frequently than in Tay-Sachs disease. In type B there is visceral involvement; the central nervous system and thus the retina are spared.

The other diseases listed are all extremely rare.

Question 39

1. List five abnormalities.
2. What is the diagnosis?

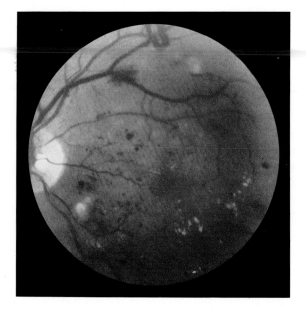

Answer to question 39

1. (a) Microaneurysms.
   (b) Haemorrhages (intraretinal and nerve fibre layer).
   (c) Cotton wool spots.
   (d) Venous loop.
   (e) New vessels at the disc.
2. Proliferative diabetic retinopathy.

The onset of proliferative diabetic retinopathy is preceded by increasing retinal ischaemia. The characteristic signs of pre-proliferative diabetic retinopathy are:

(a) Cotton wool spots (nerve fibre layer infarcts)
(b) Retinal haemorrhages (in increasing number)
(c) Venous changes (loops and beading)
(d) Arteriolar narrowing
(e) Intraretinal microvascular abnormalities (IRMA)

Intraretinal microvascular abnormalities (IRMA) are seen at the edge of areas of retinal ischaemia. They appear as bizarre vessel formations within the retina. Whether they represent attempts at neovascularisation or remodelling of pre-existing capillaries is unclear. Patients with pre-proliferative retinopathy require close ophthalmological follow up. Panretinal photocoagulation is performed at the first sign of proliferative change.

Question 40

A 35-year-old man had an episode of loss of vision in the right eye 3 years ago.

How would you describe the appearance of the right optic disc?

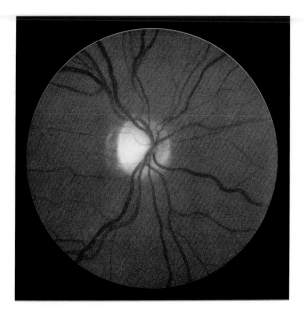

Answer to question 40

Temporal pallor.

Temporal pallor is the characteristic sign of past optic neuritis. Inflammatory and toxic conditions involving the optic nerve predominantly affect the fibres of the papillo-macular bundle. The papillomacular bundle consist of fine nerve fibres originating from the ganglion cells of the macula and passing over the temporal side of the disc to reach the centre of the optic nerve. Atrophy of these fibres results in temporal pallor.

   Optic tract lesions will cause temporal pallor ipsilaterally with nasal pallor on the contralateral side. In ischaemic optic neuropathy only part of the disc may be infarcted leading to segmental pallor.

   Temporal pallor is often misdiagnosed by those inexperienced at ophthalmoscopy, the temporal side appearing slightly paler than the nasal in health. Always ask yourself whether there is loss of neuroretinal tissue at the disc and compare the appearance in both eyes.

Question 41

1. What is the prominent ophthalmoscopic feature?
2. What is the most common cause?

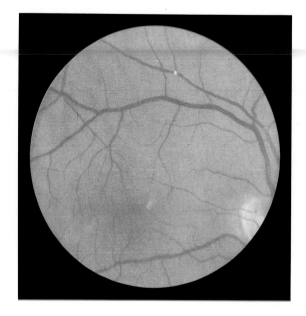

Answer to question 41

1. Cholesterol emboli.
2. Carotid artery atheroma.

Cholesterol emboli appear as glistening yellow lesions; usually at arteriolar bifurcations. They are often multiple and are located more peripherally than calcific emboli. Cholesterol emboli are mostly asymptomatic as it is uncommon for the arteriole to be totally occluded. Sometimes amaurosis fugax is the presenting symptom.

The emboli occur in showers, when an atheromatous plaque ulcerates releasing debris into the circulation. They are fragile in nature and when observed over a period of minutes can be seen to move along the retinal arterioles, indicating break up of the emboli. Other evidence of atheromatous disease (ischaemic heart disease, peripheral vascular disease and cerebrovascular disease) should be sought.

Question 42

What type of fundus is shown?

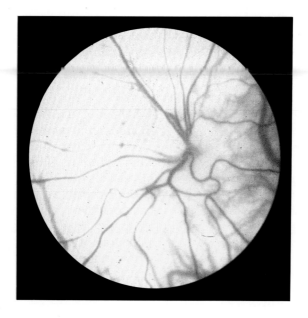

Answer to question 42

Albino fundus.

Melanin is synthesised in the retinal pigment epithelium, and by melanocytes in the choroid. There is much racial and individual variation in the amount of pigment present. In albinism there is a defect in the synthesis of melanin from tyrosine. The fundus does not develop its normal orange colouration, which allows the bizarre, ramified pattern of the choroidal vasculature to be seen beneath the retinal vessels.

Oculocutaneous albinism is an autosomal recessive condition, characterised by hypopigmentation of skin, hair, fundus and irides. They also have nystagmus, photophobia and decreased visual acuity. Melanocytes are present but contain immature melanasomes with very little melanin. Tyrosinase negative and tyrosinase positive types may be identified by incubating complete hair follicles in tyrosine; those from positives darken. The degree of pigmentation is usually greater in tyrosinase positive individuals but the vision is still poor.

Ocular albinism is a rare X-linked condition affecting the eyes only; skin pigmentation is normal. Female carriers can be identified by characteristic retinal pigmentary changes in the fundal periphery.

Question 43

A 64-year-old woman is referred from her general practioner with a fundal abnormality. Three years previously she had a partial mastectomy.

What is the most likely cause of this appearance?

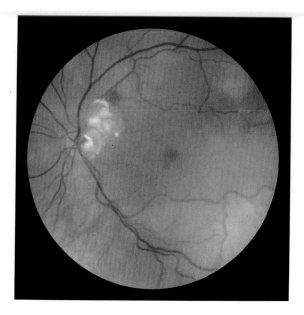

Answer to question 43

Choroidal secondaries from carcinoma of the breast.

Secondary carcinoma of the choroid is the commonest intra-ocular malignancy. They appear as pale oval patches most often at the posterior pole. The edges are indistinct, as the secondaries tend to spread through the choroid and are only minimally elevated. There may be some mottling due to clumping of the overlying retinal pigment epithelium. In this case there is a secondary visible at the optic nerve head, where it displaces the vessels. There is a larger secondary infiltrating the choroid at the inferior temporal edge of the picture. The commonest sites of primary carcinomas are the breast and lung. Renal, gut and testicular primaries have been reported. Choroidal secondaries are often bilateral. The patient usually has a previous history of malignant disease. Unless the optic nerve is invaded visual symptoms are rare. Orbital pain does occur (unlike malignant melanoma). Radiotherapy will generally induce regression. Only rarely is surgical intervention required for relief of intractable pain.

Question 44

1. Name two abnormalities.
2. What is the diagnosis?

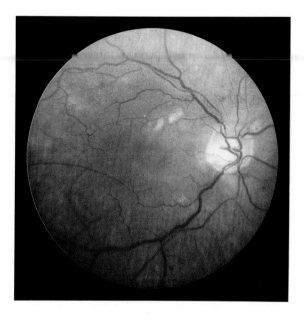

Answer to question 44

1. (a) Arterio-venous abnormalities.
   (b) Variations in arteriolar calibre.
   (c) Cotton wool spots.
   (c) Retinal haemorrhages.
2. Vascular hypertension.

There is a normal age-related change in the retinal vasculature, involutional arteriosclerosis. With age the retinal arterioles become straighter, paler, narrower and branch more acutely. These changes become evident between 50 and 60 years of age. The effects of systemic hypertension, of any cause, upon the retinal vasculature are superimposed upon these arteriosclerotic changes.

Of the many fundal signs described in hypertension some are more reliable than others. Vessel tortuosity and changes in the light reflexes from the vessels (silver and copper wiring) are subjective signs which are difficult to quantify and this limits their usefulness. Vessel narrowing and straightening do not help to distinguish hypertensive from arteriosclerotic changes and are thus less reliable in patients older than 50. More reliable signs are variation in arteriolar calibre, arterio-venous crossing changes, haemorrhages, exudates, cotton wool spots and papilloedema.

The first reaction of the retinal arterioles to hypertension is sustained spasm, sometimes described as hypertonus. In the arteriosclerotic fundus the vessels undergo patchy replacement fibrosis of their media. These areas dilate whilst healthier areas constrict. Arterio-venous (A-V) changes occur where the vessels are contained within a common adventitia, at their crossings. They consist of:

(a) Concealment of the vein beneath the artery — A-V nipping.
(b) Dilatation of the distal vein.
(c) Deviation-abrupt changes in the direction of the vein at crossings, shown in this example on the superior temporal arcade of vessels.

Question 45

A 17-year-old girl complains of sudden loss of vision in the left eye associated with a dull throbbing orbital pain aggravated by eye movements. The right fundus was normal; the left is shown.

1. What is the diagnosis?
2. What special investigation would help to confirm this diagnosis?

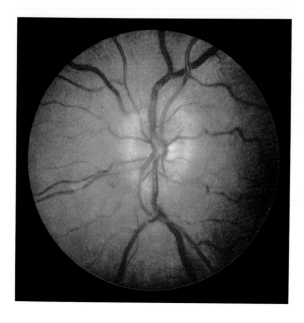

Answer to question 45

1. Papillitis.
2. Visually evoked potentials (VEP).

Optic neuritis is an inflammatory or demyelinating process involving the optic nerve. Papillitis can be regarded as an intraocular optic neuritis, i.e. distal to the lamina cribrosa. The term retrobulbar neuritis refers to the involvement of the optic nerve behind the lamina cribrosa, the disc appearing normal. Both conditions present as sudden loss of vision, which may be moderate to severe. Orbital pain is common and typically aggravated by ocular movements. There is an afferent pupillary defect (Marcus-Gunn pupil), with decreased appreciation of colour and light brightness. Increases in body temperature (e.g. hot baths, vigorous exercise) will often cause further deterioration in vision (Uhthoff's phenomenon). It is these clinical features which distinguish papillitis from papilloedema, the fundal appearances being similar. However in papillitis the optic cup is lost at an early stage, inflammatory cells spilling into the vitreous make it difficult to get the nerve head into sharp focus.This inflammatory process may extend onto the retina itself (neuroretinitis) with fine hard exudates and a macula star.

Papillitis is most common in children when it frequently follows a viral illness. There may be other features of viral encephalitis. Retrobulbar neuritis is commoner in adults. In about 50% of cases the patient will have or will develop multiple sclerosis. Of the remainder many are idiopathic, a few are caused by spread of inflammation from contiguous structures (e.g. meningitis, sphenoid sinusitis).

Visually evoked potentials are recorded by a modified EEG technique. The patient is presented with a stimulus either a single flash of light or an alternating checkerboard. Multiple recordings are made and computer averaging used to separate out the visually evoked responses. In optic neuritis there is delay in the evoked response which persists after the recovery of vision.

Question 46

A 26-year-old male was admitted to hospital following a
head injury. He was conscious and well orientated; the
overnight observations remained stable. He had a history of
previous cosmetic squint surgery. This is the appearance of
his left optic disc; the right disc was entirely normal.

What is the diagnosis?

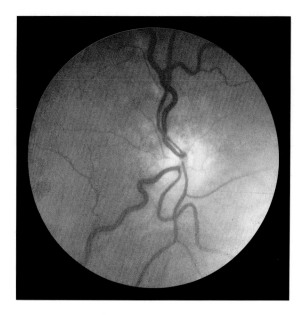

Answer to question 46

Unilateral optic nerve hypoplasia.

Optic nerve hypoplasia is a hereditary condition which may
be unilateral or bilateral. It usually occurs sporadically, but
has been reported with maternal diabetes mellitus and drug
usage (lysergic acid diethylamine, quinine, and anti-
convulsants). The nerve head is small with a peripapillary
yellowish, mottled halo approximately the size of the normal
disc. The vessels are tortuous. There is thinning of the nerve
fibre layer with a depleted number of ganglion cells. The
halo is produced by the RPE extending over the lamina
cribrosa. Presentation is usually with a childhood squint or
with nystagmus. Vision is usually reduced to around 6/36 in
affected eyes.

Optic nerve hypoplasia is associated with dysplasia of the
septum pellucidum and hypopituitarism. New cases should
have a CT scan and be followed up for signs of pituitary
hyposecretion.

Question 47

A 64- year-old man presents in casualty having awoken that morning to find impaired vision in his right eye. General examination was normal. The appearance of the right optic disc is shown.

1. What is the diagnosis?
2. Which systemic disease must be excluded, and how?

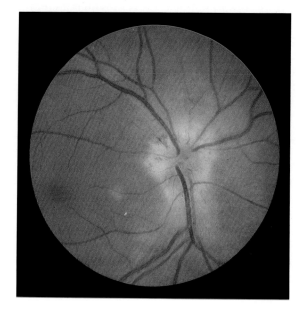

Answers to question 47

1. Anterior ischaemic optic neuropathy (AION).
2. Giant cell arteritis. Erythrocyte sedimentation rate.

Anterior ischaemic optic neuropathy (AION) presents as painless loss of vision often on waking from sleep and is an important cause of visual loss in the 45–85 year age group. The degree of visual loss is variable. Typically there is a dense inferior altitudinal field defect involving central vision. The optic disc is swollen usually (as in this example) worse in one sector. Small flame haemorrhages are seen. As the disc oedema resolves optic atrophy ensues. Arteritic and non-arteritic types must be separated, as those with giant cell arteritis need urgent high dose oral steroids to minimise the risk of bilateral involvement. Arteritis patients are usually in the 65–85 year age group, and have a history of malaise, weight loss, polymyalgia, headache, jaw claudication etc. The erythrocyte sedimentation rate is usually raised (50–120), temporal artery biopsy may confirm the diagnosis. Non- arteritic AION is associated with arterial hypertension (40%), diabetes mellitus (22%), other cardiovascular diseases (e.g. myocardial ischaemia, carotid artery disease, 23%); however in 25% of cases no systemic association is found. There is involvement of the second eye in 40% of cases after 5 years. When the second eye becomes involved the patients have optic atrophy on the original side with disc swelling on the other — the 'pseudo-Foster-Kennedy syndrome'. This is far commoner than true Foster-Kennedy syndrome due to a meningioma of the olfactory groove.

Index

acquired immunodeficiency
  syndrome, 26
age-related macular
  degeneration, 48, 52, 60
albinism, 96
amaurosis fugax, 16, 94
angioid streaks, 70
arteriosclerosis, 100

blood supply, retina, 4
blood retinal barriers, 5
Bruch's membrane, 5, 52

cherry red spot, 42, 88
chloroquine, 44
choroid, 5
choroidal naevus, 54
choroidal secondaries, 98
choroiditis see uveitis,
  posterior,
cotton wool spots, 14, 26, 32
cytomegalovirus retinitis, 26

diabetic retinopathy
  background, 40
  focal exudative maculopathy,
    40
  papillopathy, 62
  pre-proliferative, 90
  proliferative, 48, 50, 82
development ocular, 3
drusen,
  disc, 64
  macular, 46

emboli, 16, 42, 94
examination technique, 9

Foster-Kennedy syndrome, 106

fovea, 6
foveola, 5
fluorescein angiography, 50, 52

giant cell arteritis, 106
glaucoma, 24, 34

hypermetropia, 7, 38
hypertension, 14, 24, 100
hyperviscosity syndromes, 24,
  28

laser photocoagulation, 42, 50,
  52, 82
leukaemia, 22, 36

macula, 6
macular star, 14
melanoma, malignant, 80
multiple sclerosis, 102
myelinated nerve fibres, 20
myopia, 7, 84

neurofibromatosis, 68
Niemann-Pick disease, 88

ophthalmoscope, direct, 3, 7
optic atrophy, 66
optic disc, 7
  hypoplastic, 104
  myopic, 84
  tilted, 72
optic neuritis, 92, 102
optic neuropathy, 106

Index

papilloedema, 74, 86
papillitis, *see* optic neuritis
phakomatoses, 68
photoreceptors, 3
pseudopapilloedema, 38

senile macular degeneration,
　　see age-related macular
　　degeneration
Sturge-Weber syndrome, 68
systemic lupus erythematosus,
　　32

retinal artery occlusion, central,
　　42
retinal detatchment
rhegmatogenous, 84
　serous, 52, 54, 80
　tractional, 48
retinal pigment epithelium
　　(RPE), 3
retinal haemorrhages, 30
retinitis pigmentosa, 18
retinal vein occlusion
　branch, 56
　central, 24
Roth spots, 21, 36

Tay-Sachs disease, 88
tigroid fundus, 78
toxoplasmosis, 58, 76
tuberose sclerosis, 68

uveitis, posterior, 58, 76

visually evoked potentials, 102
von Hippel-Lindau syndrome,
　　68